YOU KNOW IT'S TIME FOR A SECOND OPINION WHEN . . .

THE OFFICIAL INSTRUCTION BOOK FOR HOW
<u>NOT</u> TO CHOOSE YOUR DOCTOR

by
W. Asbury Stembridge, Jr.

Illustrations by Jason Smith
Copy Editing by Melinda Burdette

Published by
TRIPLE C PRODUCTIONS
A subsidiary of Stembridge Investments, Inc.
132 Saddle Run Court
Macon, GA 31210

Copyright © 1995 by W. Asbury Stembridge, Jr.
Illustrations copyright © by Jason Smith

All rights reserved. No part of this book may be reproduced in any form or by any means without the written permission of the Publisher, excepting brief quotations used in connection with review written specifically for inclusion in a magazine or newspaper.

Printed in the United States of America

Library of Congress Catalog Number 95-90347

Stembridge, W. Asbury.
You know it's time for a second opinion when—*W. Asbury Stembridge, Jr. Macon, Ga.:*
Triple C Productions, 1995
p. cm.
ISBN 0-9646384-0-1

1. Physicians—Humor. 2. Medicine—Humor   I. Title.

R705.S84 1995   610.92

QBI95-20347

FORWARD

Helen, my wife, has strongly encouraged me to keep the day job while writing jokes. And that's fine with me. I hope my boss agrees. Working with physicians as the Director of Physician Services and Recruitment for the Medical Center of Central Georgia has a ton of benefits and equally as many pressures. The greatest stress reliever I have is looking straight into the fiery eyes of a screaming doctor and thinking of a good joke. The doctor is never the butt of the joke. I can't think that fast. But, I love to see the look on his or her face when I start smiling, almost laughing, for no apparent reason right in the middle of a vein popping tantrum. I don't get rattled. I stay confident. Who can stay angry at you for doing a good job and maintaining a good sense of humor?

I once heard the famous singer/song writer, Billy Joel, say something to the effect that song writing while on tour often led to an album of songs about life on the road. You are too focused about the trials and tribulations of traveling that your mind can't explore other areas of song writing. I find I have been influenced by that phenomenon. Doctors are terribly interesting with minds that are amazingly complex. Their stories of medical school, residency, trauma call, politics, office practice, government intervention, etc. keep me enthralled for countless hours. It is no wonder that when a joke enters my head, it usually follows some extraordinary encounter I have just had with a physician. Like the time I learned the neurosurgeons had a white rat laboratory in a local law school. Immediately, I figured, GREAT! A rat lab in a law school. I guess the docs wanted the rats to feel at home.

It quickly became evident that a combination of my interesting work and offbeat hobby would soon become partners in a joint venture of sorts. Some hospital administrators may call it a bastardized vertical integration. That's too serious. I call it fun. And because, I have never met one doctor in Macon or Central Georgia that fit the characterizations that follow, I guess I'm safe. However, in this confusing time of healthcare reform, managed care, and dwindling Medicare funds, you can use this little book as a checklist to prevent the possibility of going into a liposuction procedure and coming out like a California Raisin.

W. Asbury Stembridge, Jr.

SPECIAL ACKNOWLEDGMENTS

In 1990, I created a comedy club as annual fund raiser for the Bibb county (Macon, Georgia) unit of the American Heart Association called "Live At The Cardiac Cafe". Below is a list of the comedians who traveled from L.A. to Macon to help me out and thereby inspired me with their talents, creativity, and desire to live most anywhere other than L.A.

Jeff Altman - The first comedian to hit our stage. He is the most gentile and philanthropic celebrity I have ever met. His friendly personality and desire to help continue to amaze me.

Dave Coulier - We ate grits at a Waffle House near the Atlanta Airport and talked about golf, hockey, and roller blading. I found out then comedians are usually real people.

Blake Clark - The native Maconite who returned home twice to host the "Cardiac Cafe". He has more guts than I could ever imagine. He, Sharon, and their oldest son, Travis, packed all their belongings and headed to L.A. to be a star. And he is succeeding.

Pam Stone - The second Georgia native. Later she became a Club Comedian of the Year. When she agreed to visit the "Cardiac Cafe", her manager told me to rent a limo because Pam is over six feet tall and needed room to stretch out. We've had a limo every year since. Is this a great country or what?

Mark Curry - The first "Cardiac Cafe" veteran to get a sitcom after appearing in Macon. I believe we helped launch him to stardom. Appearing with Pam Stone, we had the world's tallest comedy show.

Jeff Foxworthy - Another Georgia asset. What a down home guy. Our first Club Comedian of the Year. His redneck jokes gave me the inspiration for this book. He deserves a world of success. It's great when I call him in L.A. and he answers the phone without asking me who I am.

James Gregory - The Funniest Man in America, and darn well deserving of the title. All he has to do is walk on stage and the audience begins complaining of facial discomfort and side aches from laughing too hard. And he does it without moving away from Marietta, GA.

George Wallace - The largest comedian in the world. If he wasn't so funny, you'd think he could crush you like an over-ripe peach. Another product of Georgia and the most recent Club Comedian of the Year. I believe I see a trend here.

Dennis Wolfberg (deceased)—Easily, the most intelligent comedian I have ever met. He was also a Club Comedian of the Year. On the limo ride to Macon, he wanted to stop and see the birthplace of Little Richard. The driver drove for several minutes, pulled in front of a rundown shack in Pleasant Hill, and gave us a two minute life story of Richard Penniman. Six months later, I learned it was all a sham because the driver had no idea that Little Richard grew up about two blocks away. Dennis, I wanted you to return to Macon so I could take you to the right house. You died before I could get you back. We all miss you.

Etta Mae - What a great character actress. She is the only comedian I would call in L.A. and find out she was baby-sitting her manager's kids. And she says she hates kids. I know better.

Anthony Griffith - When Anthony, a wonderful black comedian, did an impression of Jimmy Stewart in *"It's A Wonderful Life"*—colorized, he killed the Macon crowd. He came to Macon with only twenty-four hours notice after our headliner became ill. I had an ulcer. I should have never worried.

Ritch Shydner - A true gentleman with more material than a decade of "Saturday Night Live". He likes my name and first thought I was a blue blooded socialite. If you ever hear him use it in a set, call me. I'll need the royalties.

Gary Mule Deer - Because he wanted to play golf the day of the show, I got to play on the most exclusive course in Macon. Comedy has its rewards. He's probably the driest, most offbeat comedian I have ever met. I wish I could think like that.

Jerry Farber- In my opinion, he is the king of the one liners. He makes it hard for his audiences to breathe because there is no time between setups and punchlines. Another Atlanta product whose musical talents make him one of the greatest all around performers in the business.

Brian Regan - He is my kind of comedian because he is a former college football player, a golfer, and a Floridian. With that kind of background, his ego was trained years ago to never get in the way of his success. He is the first comedian to donate his fee back to the "Cardiac Cafe". Watch for him to be your next Club Comedian of the Year.

Bob Nelson - He is the first comedian I ever wanted to appear at the "Cardiac Cafe". It took six years to get him. In the words of my good friend, Henry Davis, he is the best character actor since Red Skelton and has adopted those same Christian beliefs. What a rare find in the business.

To two guys who have yet to appear at the "Cardiac Cafe", Jeff Justice and Grant Turner. Jeff taught me comedy in his comedy workshoppes in Atlanta. It took him two times. I also learned right quickly not to take myself seriously and keep the day job. I hope my hobby pays off, though. I still owe him some tuition fees.

I first met Grant through his cousin in Macon, Frank Green. Without even meeting me, Grant agreed to do a Children's Hospital benefit in Macon. Now, he's done two without asking for a dime. He and his lovely wife, Lynn, have a beautiful family and home in the mountains of western North Carolina. That's where success can take you.

DEDICATION

*Just in case this is the only book I ever publish,
I need to dedicate it to everyone who has been extremely supportive.*

Helen, my wife of more years than she wants the world to know (I hope distribution goes that far). She tells me right up front, "I am not a good audience for you to try new stuff. But enough about our love life, have you written any new jokes?"

Laura, my nine year old daughter, who thinks being the subject of some of my stand up material is funny now. Wait till she has her first date and the boy has to listen to every joke I have.

Asbury, III, my nine month old son, who laughs as soon as I enter his room. Now, that's a great audience.

Charlotte and Asbury, my parents, who have guided me morally, financially, and lovingly for almost forty years. Now, as they are helping me finance this book, they are paying for my promise not to join a rock band in Cordele, Georgia in 1970.

Warren, Laurel, and Ben; my brother, sister-in-law, and nephew. Both of them work with the government. They tell all their friends, "Trust us. We're with the government." Its not original, but they've sold more of my books than the distributors.

You know it's time for a second opinion when . . .

℞ You have an appointment with your doctor, and he's there, waiting.

℞ Your proctologist's medical instruments say "Black & Decker".

℞ The logo on your doctor's medical school diploma is from Milton Bradley.

℞ Your plastic surgeon was named Physician of the Year by the Federal Witness Protection Program.

You know it's time for a second opinion when . . .

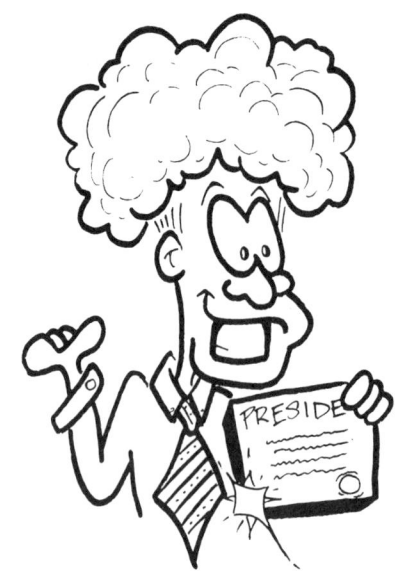

℞ Your doctor displays his plaque as president of "The Hair Club for Men".

You know it's time for a second opinion when . . .

℞ Your doctor's Christmas tree is strung with gallstones.

℞ Your doctor, in treating your severe case of the hiccups, tells you to lay down, close your eyes, and imagine your parents having sex.

℞ Your doctor calls your urinalysis appointment the 10:00 Tee time.

℞ Your doctor says forget about filing an insurance claim, just co-sign the note on his Studabaker.

You know it's time for a second opinion when . . .

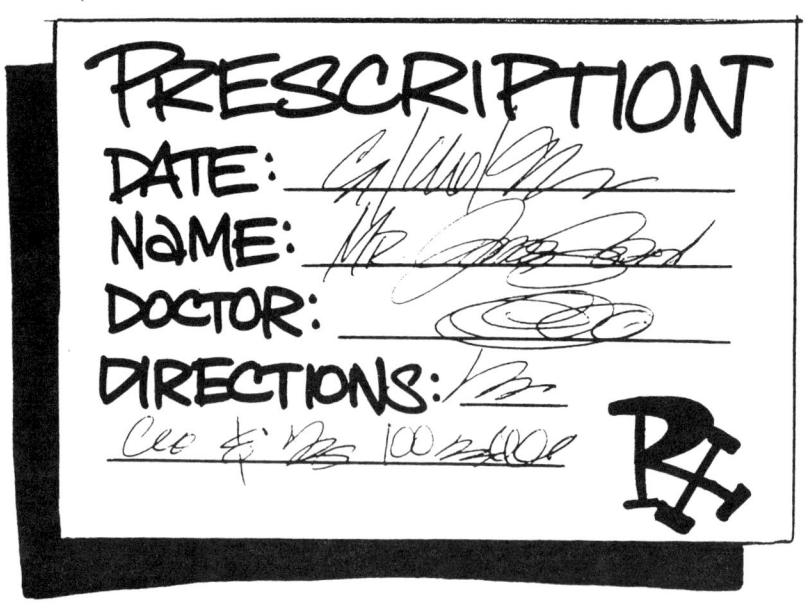

℞ Your doctor's handwriting is often confused with earthquake siesmographs.

You know it's time for a second opinion when . . .

℞ Your doctor keeps his stethoscope in ice just to watch your nipples pop out.

℞ Your doctor has a phone number for his cellular callers - *IOU.

℞ Your doctor is often called defendant.

℞ Your doctor brings a chalkboard into your exam room and tries to sell you on Amway.

You know it's time for a second opinion when . . .

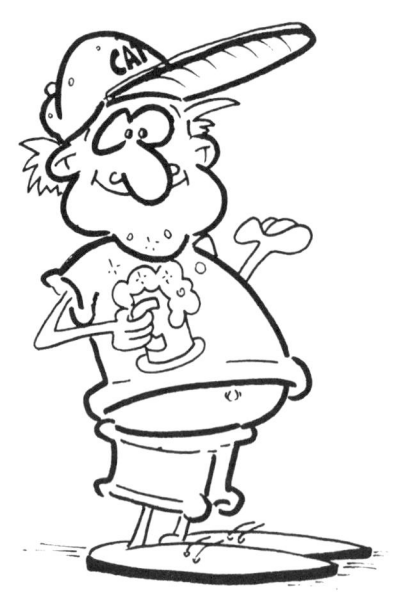

℞ Your doctor finds your beer gut is related to a skin condition - your redneck.

You know it's time for a second opinion when . . .

℞ You ask your psychiatrist to help you find your inner child and he tells you to buy an ad on a milk carton.

℞ You ask your doctor to play golf, but it's his weekend shift at Wal-Mart.

℞ Your doctor prescribes medicine for his secretary's computer virus.

℞ Your doctor's tongue depressors say "Compliments of Hart's Mortuary".

You know it's time for a second opinion when . . .

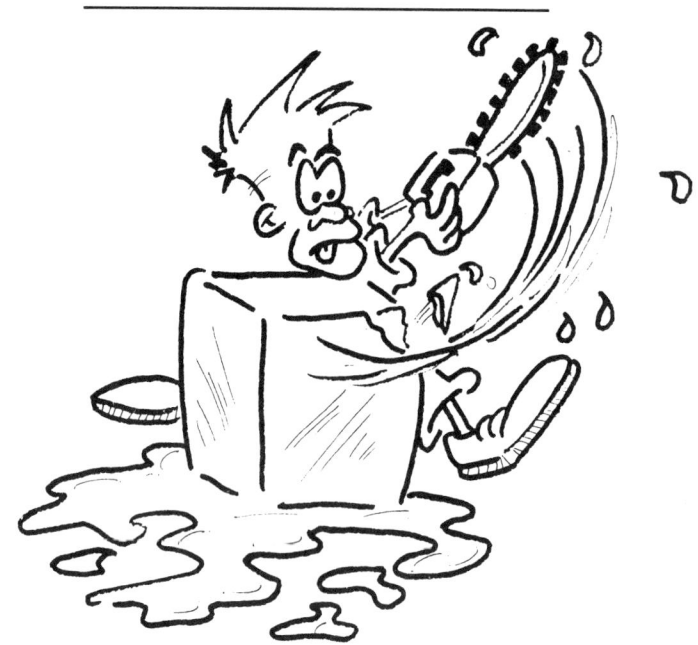

℞ Your doctor has a hobby of carving ice sculptures with a chainsaw and his most famous piece is an exact duplicate of your appendix.

You know it's time for a second opinion when . . .

℞ Your doctor says your backache is from kidney stones, your stomach ache is from gall stones, and your ear ache is from The Rolling Stones.

℞ Your gynecologist calls a local lesbian club "The Sterile Environment".

℞ Your doctor's accent is so thick, you can't understand whether you are suffering from memory loss or mammary loss.

℞ Your urologist can't make the appointment but says his wife can fill in for him because she majored in small animal husbandry.

You know it's time for a second opinion when . . .

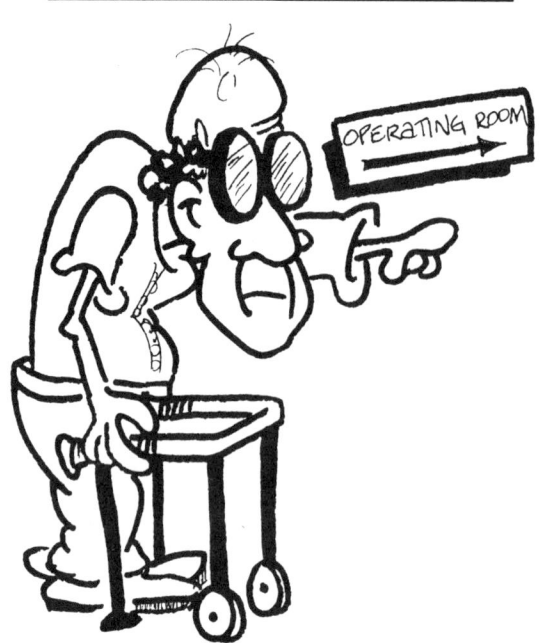

℞ Your orthopedic surgeon uses a walker.

You know it's time for a second opinion when . . .

℞ Your doctor provides you the test results from your physical and happily states you'll live to be as old as the magazines in his waiting room.

℞ Your surgeon says you have to rush right back to surgery because he has looked everywhere and still can't find his Rolex.

℞ Your doctor's medical school fraternity letters were CYA.

℞ Your doctor has an autographed picture that reads, "We won't let the next one slip away. Sincerely, Dr. Kervorkian".

You know it's time for a second opinion when . . .

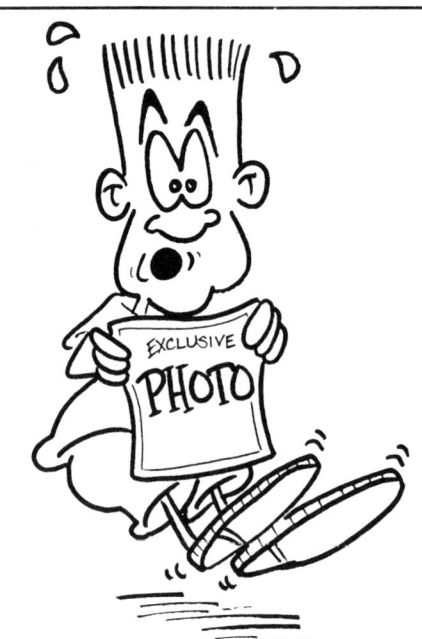

℞ You ask your doctor for an appetite suppressant and he gives you a nude photograph of Saddam Hussein.

You know it's time for a second opinion when . . .

℞ You discover the world's three most famous buses are John Madden's Cruiser, Charles Kuralt's On-The-Road, and your doc's medical school.

℞ Your doctor's rubber hammer is autographed by Tonya Harding.

℞ Your doctor's bill collector is named "Corleone".

℞ Your doctor swears he's an accomplished musician on the internal organ.

You know it's time for a second opinion when . . .

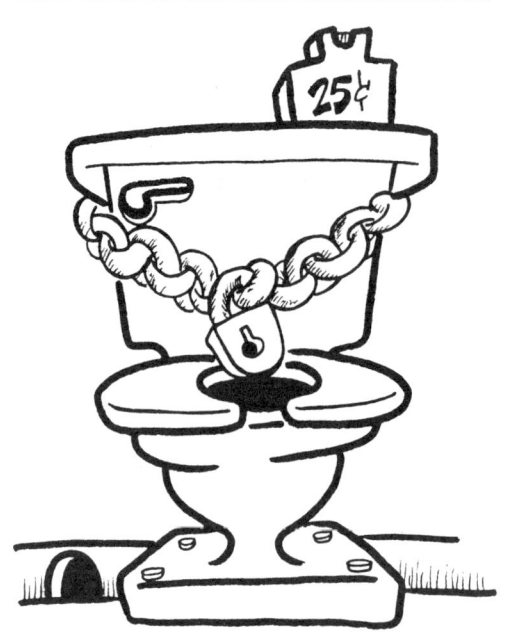

℞ Your doctor asks you for a urine sample and he has coin operated toilets.

You know it's time for a second opinion when . . .

℞ During your physical, your doctor says, "Turn your head and sing 'You Gotta Hold On Me'".

℞ Your boss asks the company psychiatrist for references and he lists Sally, Phil, and Oprah.

℞ Your doctor has a Pabst Blue Ribbon logo on his surgical mask.

℞ Your gynecologist laughs when you tell him you're wearing white at your wedding.

You know it's time for a second opinion when . . .

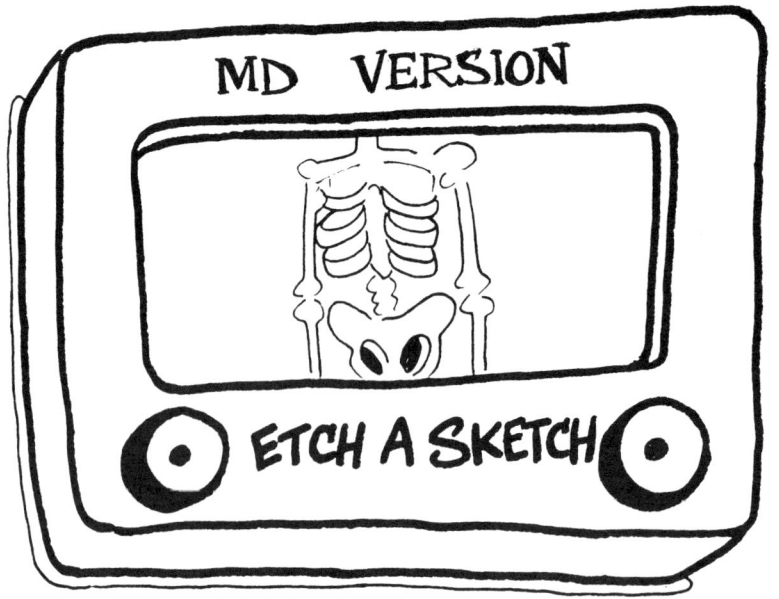

℞ Your doctor's X-Ray machine was made by Etch A Sketch.®

You know it's time for a second opinion when . . .

℞ Your obstetrician gets all expenses paid trips to London for every 50 leads he gives the Baby Book of the Month Club.

℞ Your doctor uses Whoopee cushions for breast implants.

℞ Your doctor has a hobby as a kid's party clown and makes balloon animals from penile implants.

℞ Your doctor's nurses have a tip jar on the desk.

You know it's time for a second opinion when . . .

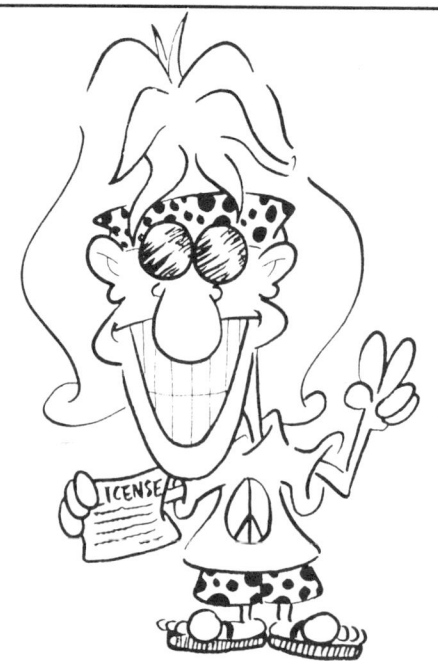

℞ Your doctor's drug license was approved by the Grateful Dead.

You know it's time for a second opinion when . . .

℞   Your doctor has any of these initials after his name: D.D.T., D.O.A., or S.O.L.

℞   Your doctor's medical school diploma has a flip side for the English translation.

℞   Your doctor's medical school yearbook says he was voted "Most Likely to be Elected to Congress... in El Salvador."

℞   Your doctor is certified in gastroeconomics -- one who charges you until you puke.

You know it's time for a second opinion when . . .

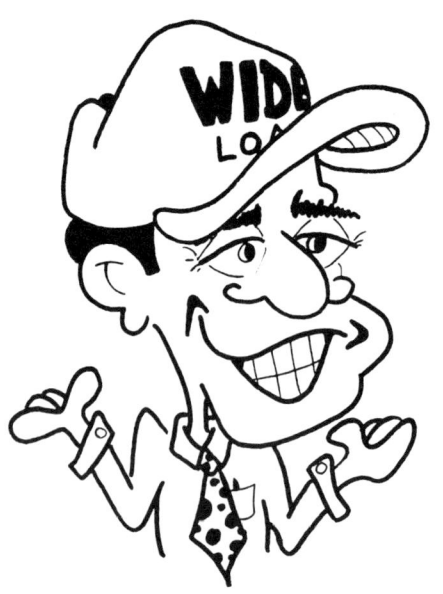

℞ The nurses give your doctor a baseball cap to match his ego that reads "Wide Load".

You know it's time for a second opinion when . . .

℞ Your doctor thinks the Pillsbury doughboy has a yeast infection.

℞ Your doctor offers to go double-or-nothing on your bill if you can find your own hernia.

℞ You prepare for your gynecological exam by placing your feet in the stirrups and the doctor plays the trumpet fanfare from the Kentucky Derby.

℞ Your doctor visits your son's eighth grade biology class and refers to the sperm's search for the egg as Where's Waldo.

You know it's time for a second opinion when . . .

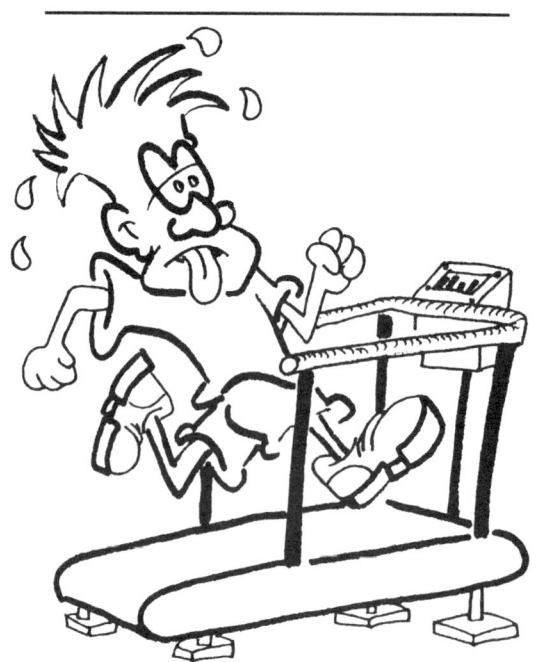

℞   Your doctor keeps you on the treadmill until your check clears.

You know it's time for a second opinion when . . .

℞   Your plastic surgeon's office has a connecting suite to Glamour Shots.®

℞   Your doctor is retired from the Navy and his eye chart is in morse code.

℞   Your orthopedic surgeon can't remember the words after, "The foot bone's connected to the ankle bone. The ankle bone's connected to the..."

℞   You're postive your physician's office manager is Natasha with the Gorgeous Ladies of Wrestling.

You know it's time for a second opinion when . . .

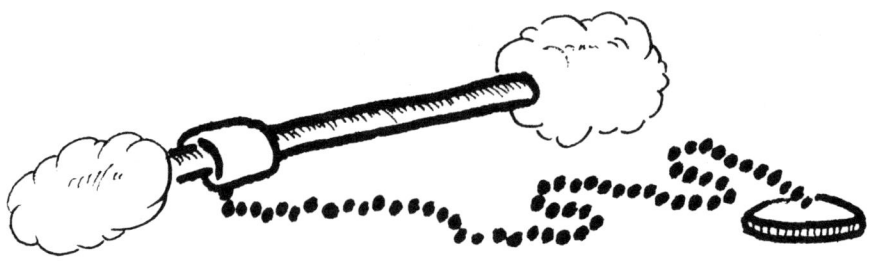

℞ Your doctor's cotton swabs are on chains like bank pens.

You know it's time for a second opinion when . . .

℞   Your doctor's telephone answering machine says, "Thank you for calling, but if you're uninsured, we're uninterested."

℞   Your doctor thinks Gluteus Maximus is a Greek hero.

℞   Your pediatrician calls your son's circumcision "trimming the pig-in-a-blanket."

℞   In your pre-natal birth classes, your doctor tells expectant fathers that afterbirth is nothing more than a Maalox moment gone bad.

You know it's time for a second opinion when . . .

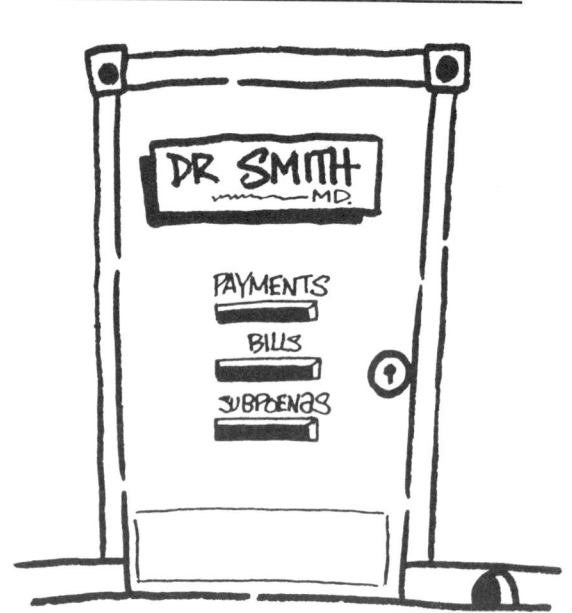

℞ Your doctor's door has 3 slots: "Payments," "Bills," and "Subpoenas."

You know it's time for a second opinion when . . .

℞ Your doctor loves politics and swears that in every election since 1964, he has voted Hippocratic.

℞ Your young doctor invites you to her wedding and her crystal pattern is the Lighthouse glass at Red Lobster.

℞ Your doctor is accused of a drive-by tetanus shot.

℞ In a moment of spiritual revelation, your doctor tries to rid your body of disease by smearing your face with blue and orange paint and yelling WAR EAGLE!

You know it's time for a second opinion when . . .

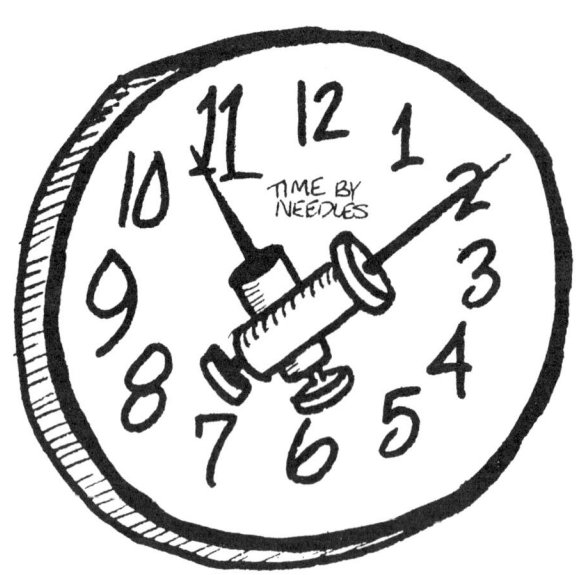

℞   The hands on your doctor's wall mounted clock are hypodermic needles.

You know it's time for a second opinion when . . .

℞ Your doctor thinks Hemlock is a chastity belt for men.

℞ Your doctor's pager goes "QUACK, QUACK, QUACK!"

℞ Your doctor's goal in life is to learn the lyrics to "Louie, Louie".

℞ Your doctor runs a special promotional offer of four Braves tickets for every vasectomy.

You know it's time for a second opinion when . . .

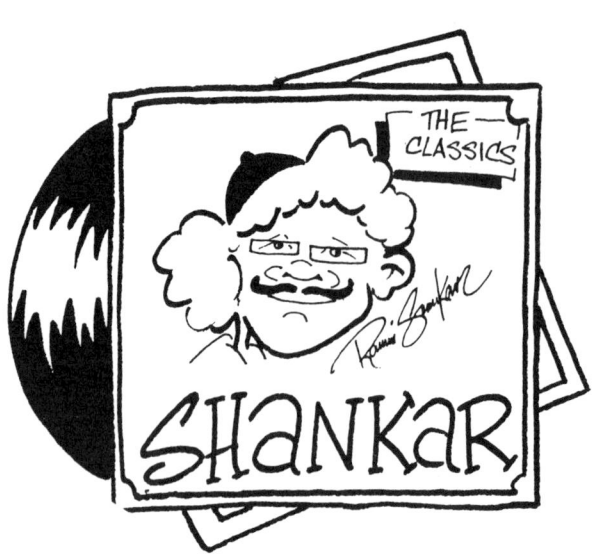

℞   You ask your doctor if he likes country music and he shows you his autographed albums of Ravi Shankar.

You know it's time for a second opinion when . . .

℞ Your orthopedic surgeon recommends shoulder surgery -- not to improve your golf game but because he needs a good caddy.

℞ Your gastroenterologist feels your flatulence problem can be traced to the Big Bang Theory.

℞ Your psychiatrist declines to use ink blots as tests but chooses cartoons from "The Far Side".

℞ Your doctor is the creator of the new television show, "America's Funniest Hernias".

You know it's time for a second opinion when . . .

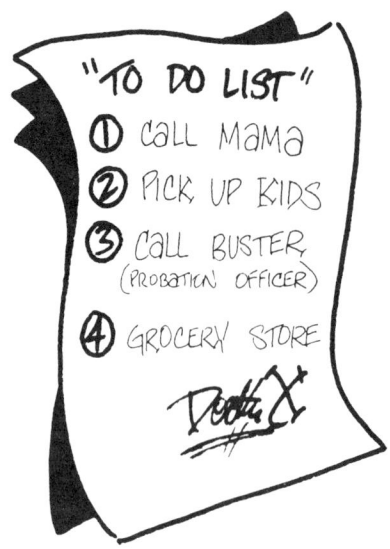

℞ Your doctor's "To Do" list includes calling his probation officer.

You know it's time for a second opinion when . . .

℞ Your doctor has a wall-mounted bronzed stethoscope with small engraved plates marking each one of his successful malpractice defenses.

℞ Your doctor's surgery bill is the showcase package on <u>THE PRICE IS RIGHT</u>.

℞ Your three family members catch the flu, and your doctor yells, "Hat Trick!"

℞ Your doctor uses the Rodney King video as a training film for testing reflexes.

You know it's time for a second opinion when . . .

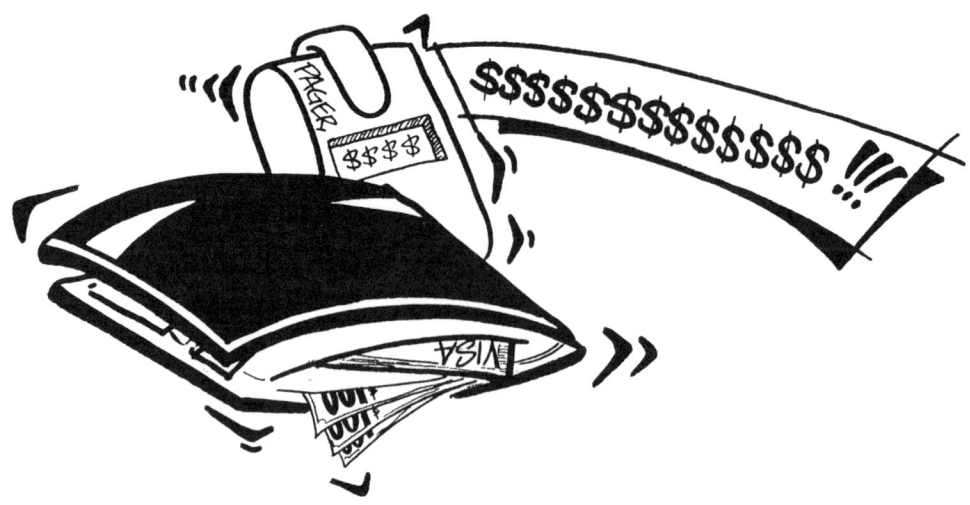

℞ Your doctor has a unique pager that doesn't beep or vibrate. It just inflates his wallet.

You know it's time for a second opinion when . . .

℞ As a medical student, your doctor earned his tuition selling fertilizer made from stool samples.

℞ Your surgeon, who is scheduled to remove your gallbladder, supplements his income as the TV spokesman for Kentucky Chicken Gizzards.

℞ Your cardiologist gives his patients $25.00 Christmas gift certificates for Varsity onion rings.

℞ You have difficulty breathing in your doctor's office when down from the ceiling drops yellow oxygen masks from Eastern Airlines.

You know it's time for a second opinion when . . .

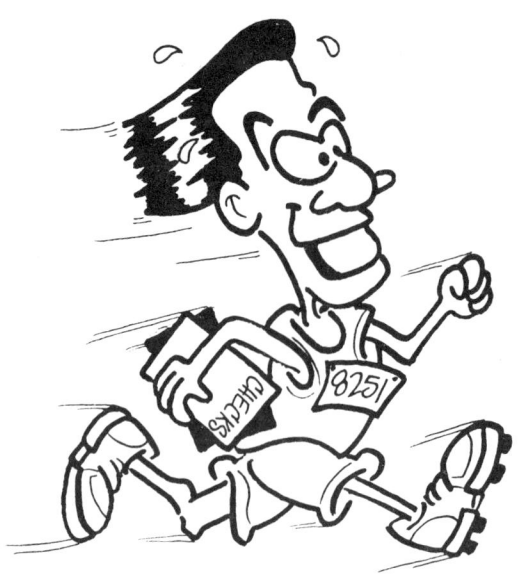

℞ You ask your doctor for an exercise program and he hires you as a runner delivering his alimony checks.

You know it's time for a second opinion when . . .

℞ Your doctor has a bumper sticker on his Lexus that reads, "A bad day golfing is better than a good day removing polyps."

℞ Your doctor's medical degree is from Pro State University.

℞ Your doctor refers to the bimbos sitting at the nightclub bar as stool samples.

℞ Your doctor sells ad space on his exam table paper.

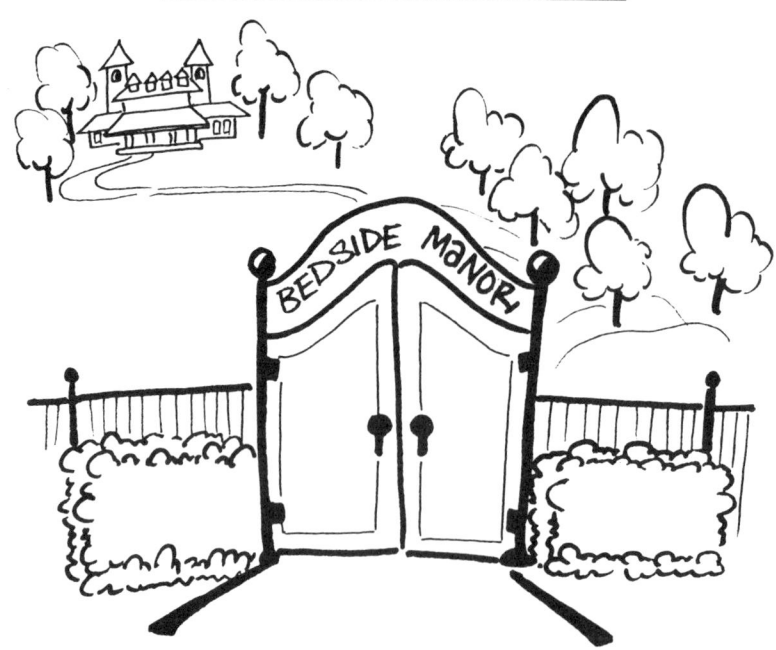

You know it's time for a second opinion when . . .

℞   Your doctor's insurance forms have coupons for Domino's.

℞   Your doctor's office has numerous posters and flyers stating, "Have you seen this child?" They're not lost. They owe him money.

℞   You think your surgeon performs the Catholic genuflect just before your case but actually his hand is asleep.

℞   Your doctor has a sign in the operating room that reads, "How's my surgery? Dial 1-800-LAWSUIT."

You know it's time for a second opinion when . . .

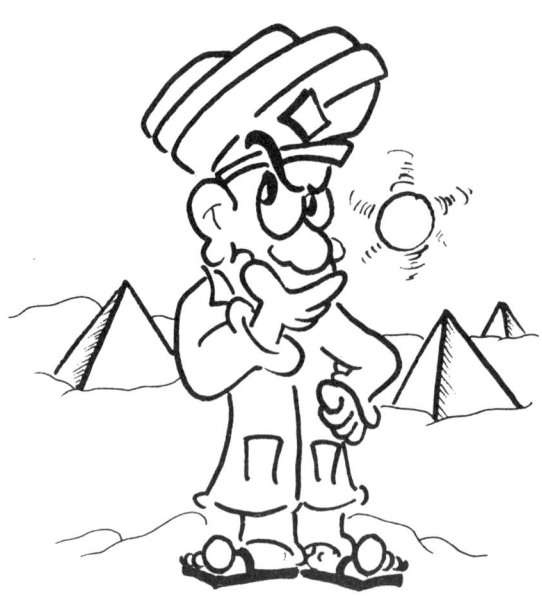

℞   Your doctor thinks all chiropractors come from Egypt.

You know it's time for a second opinion when . . .

℞   You ask your doctor for some anti-depression drugs and he gives you pills that look like Fred, Barney, and Dino.

℞   You ask your obstetrician for educational material on amniocentesis and he gives you a book on famous Clingons in Star Trek.

℞   Your doctor tells you hypochondria is nothing to bitch about.

℞   Your surgeon removes three feet of your best friend's intestine and within 24 hours opens a bait and tackle shop.

You know it's time for a second opinion when . . .

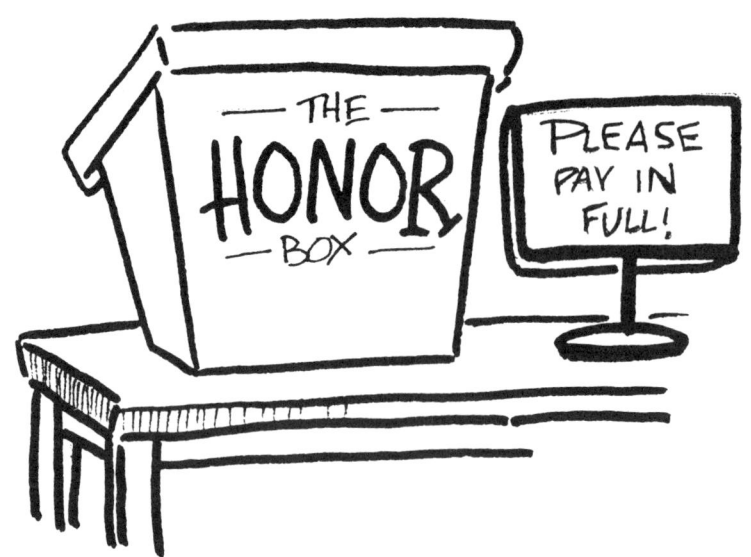

℞ You pay your doctor's bill in an honor box.

You know it's time for a second opinion when . . .

℞ Your doctor was the third guy from the left in the Village People.

℞ You ask your doctor for a motorized wheelchair and the best he can get is one with baseball cards in the spokes.

℞ Your doctor gives wedding gifts of His and Hers bedpans.

℞ As the IV fluid goes down in the bag, the picture of the centerfold model strips.

You know it's time for a second opinion when . . .

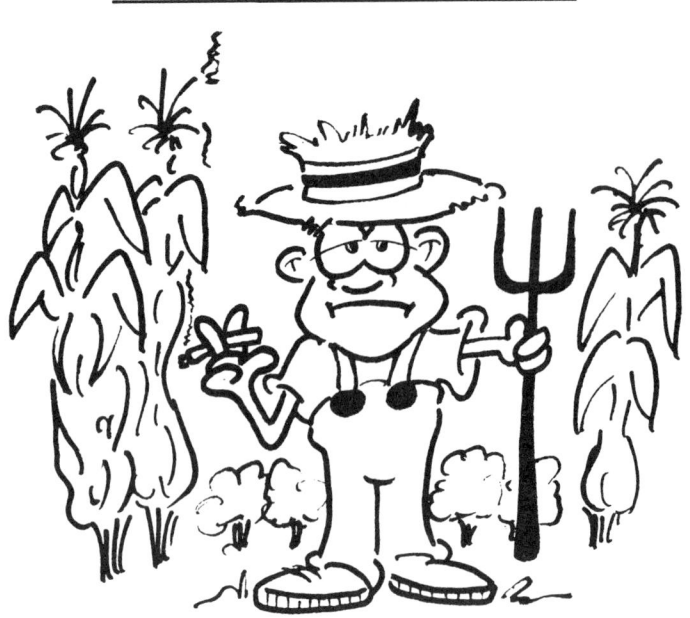

℞ You ask your doctor for a patch to stop smoking and he puts you to work in his vegetable garden.

You know it's time for a second opinion when . . .

℞ Your doctor plays Connect-the-Dots with your measles.

℞ Your spineless doctor can't give you the bad news personally, so he sends you a singing cardiogram.

℞ Your heart surgeon's idea of a great bypass is the Beltway around Washington, D.C.

℞ Your doctor has ever been interviewed by Mike Wallace of "60 Minutes".

You know it's time for a second opinion when . . .

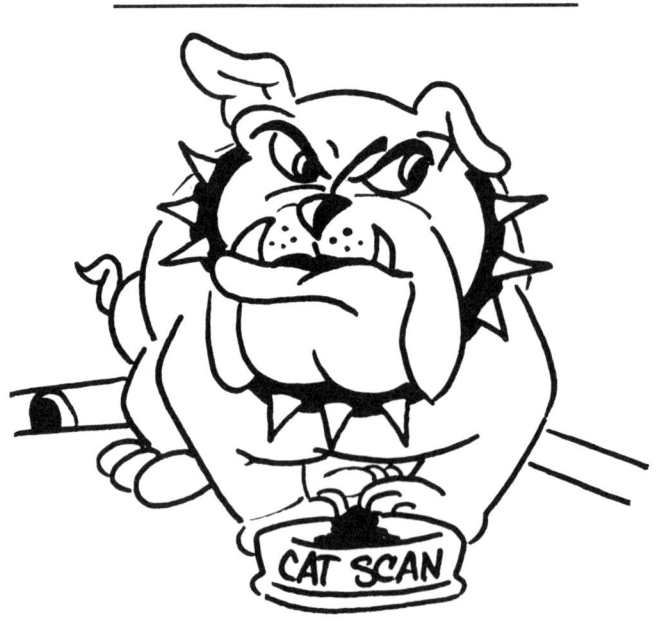

℞   Your doctor's watchdog is named CAT SCAN.

You know it's time for a second opinion when . . .

℞ The slide on your obstetrician's backyard pool is nicknamed the Fallopian Tube.

℞ Your obstetrician charges you and your husband double for treating sympathy pains.

℞ Your psychiatrist feels the only problem with biting nails is the teeth marks you leave in the sheetrock.

℞ The pacemaker your nearsighted heart surgeon plans to insert is actually a souvenir hockey puck.

You know it's time for a second opinion when . . .

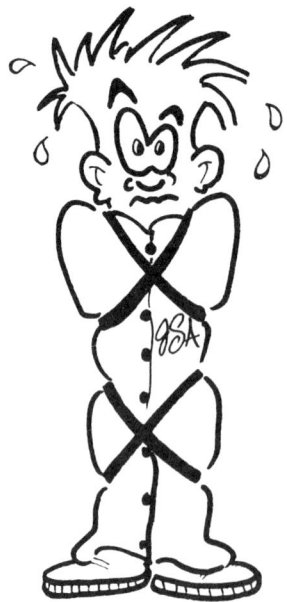

℞   Your company psychiatrist gives you a monogrammed straitjacket.

You know it's time for a second opinion when . . .

℞   Your doctor has ever appeared as an expert witness on "The People's Court".

℞   Your urologist carries two brands of penile implants -- The Pump and The Diehard.

℞   Your doctor attaches electrodes to your head while wearing an executioner's mask.

℞   During your stress test, the doctor asks you to run faster on the treadmill because the nurses need more power for the microwave.

You know it's time for a second opinion when . . .

℞ Your doctor has the entire collection of "From Butts to Boobs: The History of Plastic Surgery" from Time-Life Video.

You know it's time for a second opinion when . . .

℞   With six electrodes strapped to your chest, your doctor asks you to hold the antenna with the tinfoil so his nurses can watch THE YOUNG AND THE RESTLESS.

℞   Your doctor's idea of a stress test is to hope his beeper doesn't go off while playing golf at Augusta National.

℞   Your doctor lets out a Jekyll & Hyde-style laugh when he rips the sticky electrode pads off your hairy chest.

℞   Your doctor's office is next to the luncheonette at J-Mart.

You know it's time for a second opinion when . . .

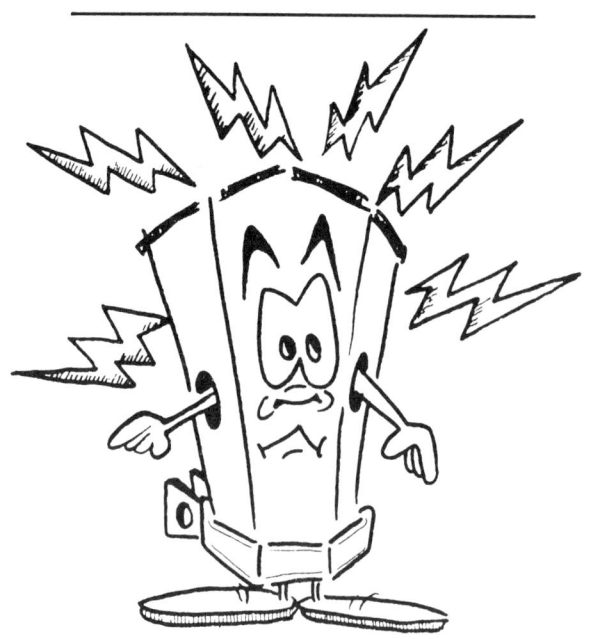

℞ Your doctor adds too much barium to your enema and you can now double as your child's night light.

You know it's time for a second opinion when . . .

℞ Your doctor's surgical cap has seven types of fishing lures.

℞ Your surgeon postpones your case because his scalpel is being held in superior court as Exhibit A.

℞ Your doctor can discount his fees if you don't feel sterilization is a necessity.

℞ Your pregnant wife's obstetrician agrees with her that it's your fault she doesn't have a thing to wear.

You know it's time for a second opinion when . . .

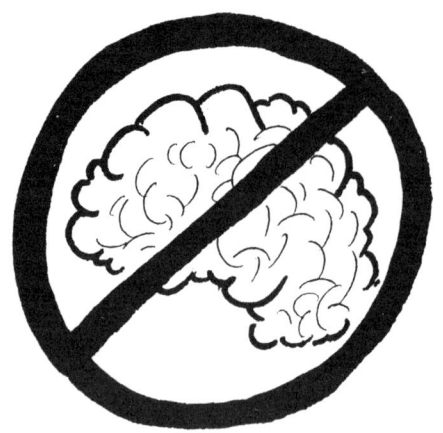

℞   Your neurosurgeon calls your case a "no-brainer".

You know it's time for a second opinion when . . .

℞   Your surgeon runs out of clamps to shut off the flow of blood and switches to Chip Clips.

℞   Your doctor thinks a paradigm shift is the overdrive on his Lamborgini.

℞   Your doctor often visits the neighborhood 7-11 to swap homeland stories with the clerk.

℞   Your psychiatrist's couch has satin sheets.

You know it's time for a second opinion when . . .

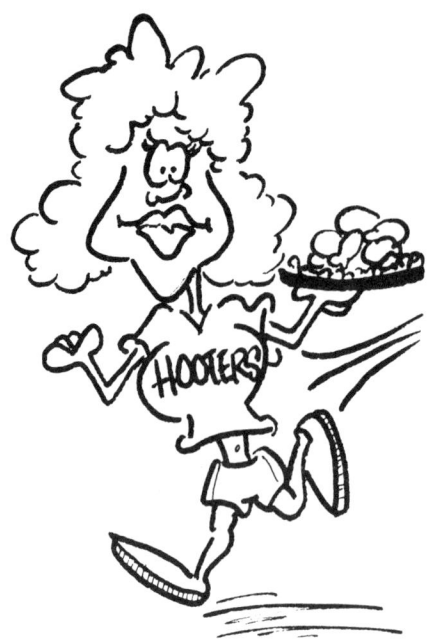

℞   Your plastic surgeon turned down the offer to become the company doctor for Hooters.

You know it's time for a second opinion when . . .

℞ Your proctologist is humming, "Take this Job and Shove It!"

℞ Your dermatologist has a restaurant called "Pizza Face."

℞ Your doctor's scrub suit says PROPERTY OF PANAMA CITY BEACH JAIL.

℞ Your doctor says there is a cheaper way than X-rays to locate your old war shrapnel -- refrigerator magnets.

You know it's time for a second opinion when . . .

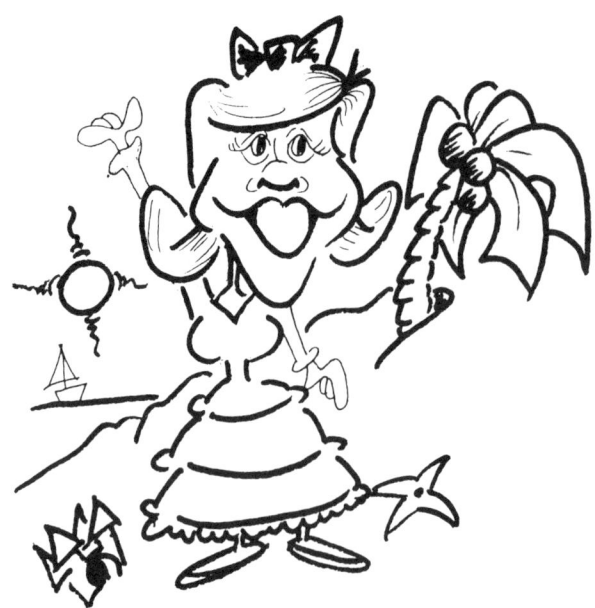

℞ Your doctor's magazines are so old, the <u>SPORTS ILLUSTRATED</u> models are wearing hoop skirts.

You know it's time for a second opinion when . . .

℞   Your doctor's partners are Dr. Howard, Dr. Fine, and Dr. Howard.

℞   Your doctor says he hasn't been able to keep a wife since he was appointed medical director of hospital affairs.

℞   Your pulmonologist can't understand why seventeen female patients have claimed sexual harrassment when he told them they have a great set of lungs.

℞   The pathology report on your mole comes back stating, "The lesion was self-contained, showed no discoloration, and tasted just like chicken."

You know it's time for a second opinion when . . .

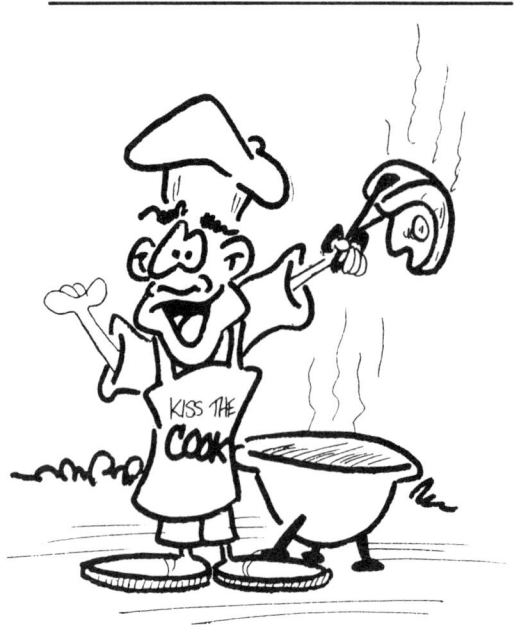

℞ Your obstetrician invites you to dinner and he uses his delivery forceps to grill your steak.